The Prison Within

by

Michael Padgett

Table Of Contents

Introduction

Throughout my five years of college life, I was plagued with constantly getting in my own way (mentally speaking), by overthinking and analyzing processes and solutions to ALL of my course to varying degrees, and even doubting my reasoning for returning to school or whether I could even be successful. The fact of the matter is that we all struggle with getting in our own way mentally. We doubt our self-worth by telling ourselves that we are flawed, not important, don't have anything to offer, and are unloved. It is these issues that are at the forefront of those seeking to self-harm or worse. Additionally, we struggle with guilt, shame, resentment, and unforgiveness, all of which are major roadblocks to discovering and living out who you were created to be. Author Mike Murdock in his book "The Law of Recognition" stated, ""You will never change your life until you change something you do daily," and that begins with reshaping your mindset, or better yet, allowing God to reshape your thinking. Our battle against the world, the enemy, and ourselves are almost always between our ears. How is your battle going? Do you find "Self" getting in the way? These are issues that I too struggle with, pose in this book with the hope of offering alternatives and tools to combat those thoughts that so often ensnare us. We were designed for so much more than we all ever realize, I included, and more times than not it is by simply not getting out of our own way intellectually speaking. The Bible says, "But we have the mind of Christ" (1 Corinthians 2:16), but how many of us forget this spiritual truth? I know I do. I hope that this book will help the reader to gain the ability to win those battle.

The Prison Within

Chapter I:

First Things First: The Soul

"Sin is very important to the soul because sin is what disintegrates the soul; it's what attacks the soul. Sin kind of is to the soul what cancer is to the body." John Ortberg

Deuteronomy 11:13 says, "And it shall be that if you earnestly obey My commandments which I command you today, to love the Lord your God and serve Him with all your heart and with all your soul." Moses highlights something in this passage that is repeated numerous times throughout Scripture (16 times), that I think some may not see, it is the distinction between the heart and the soul. Strong's Concordance defines the soul as the place of appetite, mind, desire or will, and emotion. Theologian John Ortberg is on to something when he states that sin is cancerous to the soul. Therefore, I think it best to start at the origin of sin and how it affected, or should I say infected the soul of humanity for up to and including our day. The origin of the decaying of our souls began in the Garden of Eden (Genesis 2:15-17) when God told Adam DO NOT "eat from the tree of the knowledge of good and evil, for in the day that you eat of it you shall surely die." Now, of course, Adam and Eve didn't listen to the Lord's instructions, nor do most of us at times, but they didn't die did they? Well, physically they did not die, but they were the first "Walking Dead," recorded in history. And though they would indeed go on to have children and live to a good old age, internally they were dead. That is their spirits were dead. The part of their lives that controlled their actions and motives, was alive, but the part that rightly governs the heart of mankind was dead, and that void was passed down from generation to generation until the Redeemer of our souls and Restorer of our spirit would come and pay the penalty.

In other words, the Bible makes a distinction from the physical life of mankind (the soul) and that which rightly governs the heart (the spirit). That which encompasses our mind, will, motives, and appetites are the soul. It is the striving and worrying about what the world has to offer, what is in it for me, what do others think about me, and what do I think about myself in comparison to the world. It is a skewed perspective that is selfish, self-serving, self-indulging, and ultimately self-destructive because what governs us is external, not internal. Whereas when our spirits are made alive in Christ, we look to Him for guidance, instruction, and purpose. It is where we get our value and worth. We look at how I can be selfless and helpful rather than selfish or helpless. It is where we begin to see others, as well as the self in the light of love and compassion that God created us to experience. And yet because of our corrupt nature, we need the Lord to, according to Ezekiel 36:26, "give you a new heart and put a new spirit within you," Paul like Moses, also draws out in Hebrews 4:12 about the distinction between soul and spirit, "For the word of God is living and powerful, and sharper than any two-edged sword, piercing even to the division of soul and spirit, and joints and marrow, and is a discerner of the thoughts and intents of the heart." The thoughts and intentions of the heart are directed by the thoughts and intentions of our flesh which is why Paul also states in Galatians 5:16, "Walk in the Spirit, and you shall not fulfill the lust of the flesh." That is to say, "whichever you are allowing govern your actions will be the dominant force in your life."

Of course, we know that this is easier said than done. We start well by confessing Jesus as Lord, get plugged into a good church, start reading the bible regularly and allowing the Spirit to guide as is right and true. But perhaps you have heard the adage "Good habits die hard?" An old relationship returns, we experience a disappointment or a loss, and the next thing you know we fall into the old way of thinking and doing. In other words, humans have a spirit and a soul, though the Bible makes it clear that because of our sinful nature that we are spiritually dead apart from Jesus and yet the soul continues to live on (walking dead), dictating the actions and motives of our life. The soul and the spirit are at the center of our spiritual and physical experiences, the issue then becomes, by which are we being governed.

Ultimately, the soul speaks to quality of life, it is in many places in the Bible eluded to as the biological life (Matthew 2:20, Revelation 12:11 translate soul to life/lives), and as the person (Ezekiel 18:20 translate soul to person), In essence, the soul is our humanity and the spirit becomes our connection or the inability to connect to God because apart from Jesus, the spirit is dead. While these are both interconnected, they are separable. Finally, the soul is the place of appetite, mind, will, and emotion. It is the place where think and feel, where we organize or become disorganized. It is where we focus or become distracted, where we experience pleasure or hurt energy or disappointment. It is where we become anxious, worried or experience peace and confidence.

Ultimately, it becomes a matter of what feeds those thoughts and feelings, and how we convey them. Our appetites or desires, mind, will, and emotions, whether self-indulgent or restraint, feed into how we perceive things and how we act them out. While the soul is the life in which we daily live, it is filled with corruption apart from the renewing of our spirits. Therefore, it houses a terminal disease called sin, that on our own we cannot restrain or defeat. As a result, we end up tolerating it, become accepting of it, and at a certain point become numb to its deadly consequences. It is why there is constant striving between knowing the right things to do and actually doing them, again Paul not only said as much, but he too struggled with this war within, "For the good that I will to do, I do not do; but the evil I will not to do, that I practice" (Acts 7:19). It basically comes down to what is driving our motives and actions? R. C. Sproul stated, "I cannot have God in my heart if He is not in my head. Before I believe in, I must believe that." Is it the head or the heart? And if it is the heart, has it been renewed? Or is it the head that does not operate from the mind of Christ? I have heard it said many times and in various ways that there is roughly 18 inches between heaven and hell, the distance between head and heart, or as Moses stated "heart and soul," and in the following chapters will begin to unpack each component and reveal the negative aspects that they encompass as well the results and healthier alternatives.

> *"The soul which has come into intimate contact with God in the silence of the prayer chamber is never out of conscious touch with the Father; the heart is always going out to Him in loving communion, and the moment the mind is released from the task upon which it is engaged, it returns as naturally to God as the bird does to its nest."* E.M. Bounds

Mind

"Satan target is your mind and his weapon are lies." Warren Wiersbe

Romans 12:6 (AMP) says, "Do not be conformed to this world (this age), [fashioned after and adapted to its external, superficial customs], but be transformed (changed) by the [entire] renewal of your mind [by its new ideals and its new attitude], so that you may prove [for yourselves] what is the good and acceptable and perfect will of God, even the thing which is good and acceptable and perfect [in His sight for you]." Two elements in this passage are very important to take note of. First, the word conformed. This word means "Fashioned after or having the same form as another." And two opposing competitors are seeking to form or fashion our minds to think like them, The Lord and the Devil. The Lord seeks to renew our minds to see the things of God, and the Devil uses deception to entice us with the vices of a corrupt world to attempt to shape and form our minds. In other words, Satan uses externals elements, material objects to affect change internally. The Devil, through the world, wants to change us from the outside in by pressuring, enticing, and tormenting us with shiny objects such as materialism, status, and sex. And often it is sex that is the most prominent of these shiny objects. We see it everywhere, on television, in movies, on billboards, video games, computer screens, and magazines. For example, we see a model wearing a bikini while eating a burger to promote a fast food restaurant knowing full well that she doesn't eat double cheeseburgers, and yet we are enticed to go purchase that burger because our minds have been stimulated by a shiny bead.

Sexual sin and deviance have been around since very early in humanity. It was the enticing of Delilah that would be the undoing of Sampson (Judges 16). Then there was Tamar who played the role of a prostitute to deceive Judah (Genesis 38). And who can forget about king David? He was so enticed by what he saw in Bathsheba that ultimately resulted in him committing murder (2 Samuel 11), and then tried to bury it. What was created to be a beautiful experience between husband and wife and an expression of oneness, the world has corrupted and made it into something that has destroyed marriages, families, businesses, and ministries all because the world was able to pressure from the outside the mind in order to fashion it after its kind, and ultimately corrupt the soul. It is no surprise that America is the number one exporter and consumer of pornography, and that sex trafficking is at an all-time high. By using deception, Satan attempts to draw us from the things of God to the base things of the world, and for most men it is the allure of a women which is what he did in the garden, 2 Corinthians 11:3, "But I fear, lest somehow, as the serpent deceived Eve by his craftiness, so your minds may be corrupted from the simplicity that is in Christ."

Simplicity is all too often undervalued and overlooked. I remember being in India and speaking with the young believers there and being astounded at their simplicity of thought and lifestyle. We spoke about how much of their generation is consumed with materialism and how it never seems to be enough. When I was growing up it was referred to as "Keeping up with the Jones." We see it here in the West in abundance, and never more so than when the holidays roll around or when the iPhone comes out. People are lined up around the store for hours and then proceed to stampede one another over insignificant items, and as a result, people are often injured, including the elderly and young children. It is a tragic condition of our current culture, and what's worse is that companies and advertising agencies depend on our commercialism feeding frenzies and take advantage of that by hiring Psychologists to further manipulate our minds. These, according to the Bible, operate in the futility of their minds and are surrendering to the blindness of greed (Ephesians 4:17-19). So, getting back to those young believers. They didn't dismiss the thought of what it might be like to have better things, but they said, "We do not look for the big things. If we have God, rice, and shelter it is enough, and we will praise God regardless." That is the simplicity of mind. It is not a bad thing to want to be able to enjoy a new iPhone or car or whatever, in its proper context. The issue is when we have let those things draw us away from the things of God by the deception of more is better, because the more we have the more we think we are more than we are, and that is a tactic that the enemy counts on working in his favor. This is an effort to fashion us after his corrupted image, making us worshippers of false gods and images, which is in opposition of having the mind of Christ, being fashioned in the image of God, and worshipping the one true God.

The good news is that Jesus wants to dispatch the Holy Spirit to fill, cleanse, and transform us from the inside and create an outflowing into the lives of others. The word "Transform" is where we get the word metamorphosis and is the same word used in Matthew 17 ion the mount of transfiguration. Unlike the Devil's attempt to pressuring us from the outside to affect change within, the Holy Spirit begins to affect change within that will be manifested outwardly. As a result, it changes perspective, motives, and actions because we have the Holy Spirit directing us and bringing us into unity with the mind of Christ. But without this renewing power of the Holy Spirit, we will continue to be carnally minded, which is death (Romans 8:6). Therefore, we need the transforming power of the Holy Spirit, for no one knows the mind of Jesus but the Holy Spirit. "For "who has known the mind of the Lord that he may instruct Him?" But we have the mind of Christ" (1 Corinthians 2:16). But when there's a transformation of our minds, we then can live in simplicity and contentment. When our minds are renewed, we are not shaken or moved by the things of the world, we can keep things in their proper place and appreciate the things we have versus the things that others have. As a result, we no longer waste our time, resources, or energy in pursuit of things that are unprofitable, hurtful, or harmful. We begin to look at opportunities to be the blessing instead of chasing the blessing. I often have said that we are called to be fountains of God's blessings, not reservoirs. Reservoirs tend to simply be a collection of water that unless they are stirred, will become stagnant, and stagnant water can be deadly. However, by being founts of god's blessings, we ultimately receive greater blessings.

In the end, the enemy doesn't so much have an issue with us going to church. The fact is, many of the hurts and fractured relationships have come from those in the church because the minds are still carnal (1 Corinthians 3). It is also why many begin church-hopping or stop going to church altogether. Going to church doesn't make one a true follower of Christ any more than standing in your garage makes you a car if your mentality is not transformed. Nor does he care if you are reading the Bible, remember even he knows the Bible (Matthew 4), and if we are being honest, probably better than most of us. The purpose of allowing God to transform us is to prove or to recognize as genuine after examination the things of God and thereby testify to the world the goodness of the Lord, and ultimately living out the good and acceptable and perfect will of God (Romans 12:2).

> *"If our minds are stayed upon God, His peace will rule the affairs entertained by our minds. If, on the other hand, we allow our minds to dwell on the cares of this world, God's peace will be far from our thoughts"*
> Woodrow Kroll

Will

*"According to most philosophers, God in
making the world enslaved it. According to
Christianity, in making it, He set it free. God
had written, not so much a poem, but rather
a play; a play he had planned as perfect, but
which had necessarily been left to human
actors and stage-managers, who had since
made a great mess of it."* G. K. Chesterton

Luke 22:42 says, "Father, if it is Your will, take
this cup away from Me; nevertheless, not My will, but
Yours, be done." The word "will" from the Greek,
means choice or inclination and ever since the dawn
of time, mankind has been endowed with the gift of
choice or inclination, free-will. We have been given
the ability to choose how to govern our lives in
deciding good from bad and right from wrong. Our
very moral being rests on this fact, and although the
God of all the universe created us and has numbered
the very hairs on our heads, and though He has
absolute sovereignty to dictate to us how things ought
to be without reproach, He didn't and still doesn't.
When God breathed the breath of life into Adam, He
gave him the ability to choose how he would go about

his life. He gave Adam the ability to choose for himself whether he would stay in alignment with his Creator or go off and do his own thing. He was gifted with free will, as would every generation thereafter.

The issue with free-will as with anything that we have complete discretion of is that we often misuse or mistreat it for our benefit. Free-will, like our attitudes and actions, needs to be guarded and disciplined. Very early on in a child's life, a parent discovers that the child is inclined to do whatever they want, whenever they want, and however they want. A toddler is still discovering the world and all of the fascinating objects in their path and must begin the choice whether or not they are going to listen to their parents or pursue their desires. As a parent, we wouldn't simply allow a child to eat an entire box of cookies simply because that's what they will to do. Nor would we allow that child to wander outside and into traffic because they are inclined to. Therefore, it is the parent's responsibility to guide that child into an obedient state where they are better able to govern the impulsiveness of their will to do whatever pleases them. While it is true that we have the gift of free-will, it will ultimately self-defeating and self-destructive to live a free-willing lifestyle, and therefore necessary to discipline and train ourselves to use discretion as to when and how to allow free-will to govern our actions. Truthfully, we all have a desire to be masters of our destiny, rulers of our lives, but that doesn't mean that we get to choose to do anything we want simply because we are inclined to do so, and then proclaim that we have free-will. Discretion, discipline, and reasoning should always be the order of the day.

When Jesus came to earth as a babe in a manger, He was no less the God of the universe as He was that little babe. And I am sure that as Mary was bringing up this special child, that there were moments where she had to redirect Him from doing something that most children ought not to do. But when we read Scripture, we see that Jesus submitted entirely to an attitude of obedience toward the Father. For example, John 6:38 says, "For I have come down from heaven, not to do My own will, but the will of Him who sent Me." John's gospel isn't alone with statements like this. Jesus is the Lord of all the universe, apart from Him there was nothing created (Ephesians 3:9, Colossians 1:16), He has His glory (John 17:5), and all power (Hebrews 1:3), and therefore can choose to do whatever He pleases. And yet, He chose to humble Himself in the form of humanity and become a servant of mankind by submitting to the will of the Father. So, if Jesus, who is all-powerful was willing to do that, what makes us think that we can do any less?

The fact is, we submit all the time to the will of authorities, rules, and laws. Our employers, company policies, laws of the land, and social norms. Yet for some reason when it comes down to governing ourselves from harmful and destructive habits and choices, we are not exercising our free-will in the best way possible. I remember leading a street team into one of the surrounding communities in our area and we decided to check out this park where we knew that some of the homeless population camped. As we were ministering to people, I engaged one of the park workers that happened to be there. After a few minutes of conversation, I discovered that this person was once a believer but had become disenfranchised by the hypocrisy and failures of those charged with overseeing the congregation. This individual's emotions and personal hurt were genuine, but this person's thinking that if there were a God, then why couldn't He just step in before things like this happen violates God's gift of free-will. I explained to this person that while it is true that God could step in to prevent horrible things from happening, and furthermore could have just created a population of robots that would simply honor His word and be completely submissive. However, if that were the case, then how would He know that our love and adoration for Him were genuine and not simply programmed? There is this misconception that when an individual commits their life to the Lord that they have surrendered their free-will and can no longer think for themselves. This could not be further from the truth. James 1:5 says, "If any of you lacks wisdom, let him ask of God, who gives to all liberally and without reproach, and it will be given to him." The word "Reproach" means without regret, and this is true with all of god's gifts. He does not regret giving us free-will, He IS, however, disappointed in how we use it. He desires that our wills are in alignment with His, not because He wants to control, but because He wants to bless, and this point is most evident in Luke 22:42.

Jesus had been preparing for this moment in history since Genesis 1 because as the Alpha and Omega, He knew what would eventually need to be done. The thing that I think some people miss is that although Jesus is Lord of all when He became fully man, He had to endure all the experiences of humanity, such as fear, anxiety, and despair. Yet "for the joy set before Him, endured the cross," which meant that His will and the Father's will must to come into alignment to bestow the biggest gift to the world, salvation. This meant that there had to be a little pain for a short time to experiences the blessings of heaven and was true for Jesus then it must be the same for us. All of us want the cup of suffering to be taken from us, unfortunately, because of the acts of our first parents, that is not possible. However, we can learn the will of God, begin to allow the Holy Spirit to develop that mind of Christ that is accessible, and like James 1:5, if we lack the wisdom to properly execute our free-will, ask the Father, and see if He won't give us what we need when we need it.

> "God surpasses our dreams when we reach past our personal plans and agenda to grab the hand of Christ and walk the path he chose for us. He is obligated to keep us dissatisfied until we come to him and his plan for complete satisfaction." Beth Moore

Emotions

Proverbs 29:11, "A fool vents all his feelings, But a wise man holds them back." Emotions on the surface are not the issue. Our emotions are part of God's creation in us. Our emotions are necessary for letting others know how we feel. The last thing that anyone wants, or needs is someone assuming they know how we feel or what to feel. The issue is not emotions, but how we interpret and then convey those emotions outwardly. We live in a society that promotes the expression of emotions, it is celebrated, highlighted as an expression of our true selves, and even worshipped. The problem then is that there is no filter and consequently no restrictions or rules governing how we display our emotions. The result? A society that has become emotionally fragile. This is most evident in the political clement that we find ourselves in. Because we have promoted the free expression of our emotions apart from any filter or self-regulating, families and friendships have been ripped apart because of the venom that has poured out of people's mouths as a result of not tempering their emotions. I know the damage of misplaced and misappropriated emotions can create because my occupation deals with individuals who have emotional dysregulation and as a result, behavioral disorders have developed all because we have either caved to allowing our emotions to dictate our lives, or because of the opposite end of the spectrum, suppression.

Again, emotions alone are not the issue at hand, but it is in how we understand them and then display them. The other issue that individuals struggle with is suppressing emotions because of the perception that they are wrong or would be perceived as inappropriate or offensive. The result of holding back genuine concerns and feelings is that at some point they will be displayed outwardly in some fashion. an outburst of anger and rage are some of the more common displays of suppressed emotions that are prominent, and few places more evident than during rush-hour traffic. Perhaps we've had a bad day at work, the boss or co-worker did or said something that we didn't deal with immediately or appropriately, and now we are on the freeway yelling at people, flailing our arms, and perhaps even using expletive words and/or gestures at the individual that cut us off. Now we arrive home and continue to allow our emotions to get the better of us on those who we love all because we have not learned to evaluate how we are feeling before we act them out. "A fool vent all his feelings" (Proverbs 29:11). "Our emotions are neither the most important thing about us, something to be worshiped nor are they the least important, a problem to be avoided or ignored" (Alasdair Grove- director of CCEF's School of Biblical Counseling). Unfiltered expressions of emotion and the suppression of emotions are both dangerous to us and those around us.

Emotional abuse is a very real and damaging weapon that unfortunately is prevalent across all classes, ethnicities, and cultures. Emotional abusers are those who have been abused similarly by a family member typically who hasn't learn to deal with their feelings over disappointments and failures of their own, then releases their frustrations and hurts onto someone who is vulnerable such as a spouse or children, which then becomes a cycle that turns into learned behavior and is passed onto the next generation in either becoming the abuser or allowing victimhood to take root in the form of low self-esteem and worth which only seek out those who reinforce that mindset. I remember my first trip to Nicaragua; I met an individual who was a victim of emotional abuse for decades and the result of such treatment was utter despair and hopelessness. This is not something new or rare, it is commonly more than people realize, it is the result of people not appropriately dealing with their emotions, developing healthy coping skills, and ultimately displaying those emotions in an unhealthy and self-defeating nature. Again, our emotions on their own are part of God's creation. Emotions such as joy, happiness, love, and even anger are not bad on their own. We certainly wouldn't want people assuming they know how we feel about them or the actions and situations of society, and therefore ought to be able to express our feelings openly and without judgment. It is in, however, in how we interpret them and then misappropriate or pervert them that they then become the issue. Joy becomes self-serving and misplaced, typically at the failings of another. Happiness becomes a pursuit of short-term satisfaction that eventually ceases to satisfy. Love becomes the pursuit of things or people that make us feel good about ourselves, which ends in bad habits or bad relationships. And then there's anger. Anger turns into rage, hatred, violence, and all kinds of self-destructive behaviors. While we were created to be emotional creatures, we need to learn how to not be impulsive about our emotions, we need to become more Christ-like in this area as much as anything else.

Did you know that Jesus displayed a variety of emotions while He walked the earth? For Jesus to truly live the human experience and pay the ultimate penalty that we humans rightly deserved; Jesus had to experience a range of emotions. Let us start with the fact that Jesus felt anxiety. In Luke 22:44, it says Jesus' "sweat became like great drops of blood." This condition is known as Hematidrosis and may occur when a person is suffering extreme levels of stress; for example, facing his or her death. The anxiety and weight of Jesus bearing the sins of the world was truly overwhelming. According to Isaiah 53:3, Jesus was "A Man of sorrows and acquainted with grief." Jesus felt sadness at hearing of his friend Lazarus dying and the grief of the family because He felt love for them (John 11:3), in fact, the shortest verse in the bible says, "Jesus wept," John 11:35. And finally, Jesus got frustrated and even mad. How many times did His disciples say or do something that frustrated and irritated Him? And especially Peter, who had Foot-in-mouth disease. No incident clearer than in Matthew 16 where Jesus is explaining to His team that the time is drawing near when He must fulfill His intended mission for coming to earth. The next thing you see is Peter inserting his foot by trying to prevent Jesus from completed the Father's instructions, Matthew 16:22 "Then Peter took Him aside and began to rebuke Him, saying, "Far be it from You, Lord; this shall not happen to You!" How many times have we overstepped our place and offered misplaced advice or direction? For three years Jesus had been with them, teaching, guiding, and preparing them for His eventual departing, and Peter still doesn't get it and Jesus' frustration comes out full force, "Get behind Me, Satan! You are an offense to Me" (v.23). Yeah, Jesus, the Lover of our souls, the Giver of life, gets mad. However, His anger was not misplaced or misused and is, therefore, our blueprint on how and when we allow our emotions to be displayed. He created us with our emotions and therefore knows how best to interpret and release them.

"Satan frequently either unsettles the emotions of the physical bodies of spiritual believers, or he blocks the works of the spiritual ones, or he may disturb their environments." Watchman Nee

Appetite

"Wisdom does not show itself so much in precept as in life - in firmness of mind and a mastery of appetite. It teaches us to do as well as to talk; and to make our words and actions all of a color." Lucius Annaeus Seneca

Proverbs 23:2 says, "And put a knife to your throat If you are a man given to appetite." The word "Appetite" could be replaced with passion. The thing which garners the attention of all our senses, sight, smell, sound, and taste are all affected or infected by what we allow to occupy them. Now passion isn't necessarily a bad thing if it is directed wisely and appropriately. One should be passionate about following and serving the Lord. One should be passionate about the spouse and their children. One can even be passionate about life or a meaningful occupation such as healthcare or teaching. Passion, correctly applied, can be an extremely powerful motivator. However, passion misapplied can be harmful and hurtful. Things such as the lust for unhealthy relationships or selfish pursuits of wealth, power or status at the expense of others. And the Church is not exempt from such misplaced passions.

Far too many times we hear about the fall of church leaders over sexual sins or financial failings. As one who has served in a variety of leadership roles within the church, I have seen firsthand those who pursue ministry because of the romance and recognition of it, and almost always what happens is that person becomes distracted by the symbol or status over the work which ultimately ends in some spiritual failing are drifting away from the Lord. The truth is, the ministry is not a glamorous occupation when done passionately and honestly but getting caught up in the status is a false passion, which is carnal by nature.

The Bible highlights the dangers of allowing enticing sensations to govern our motives and actions, 1 John 2:16, "For all that is in the world—the lust of the flesh, the lust of the eyes, and the pride of life—is not of the Father but is of the world." Our appetites are fed by our 5 sensations and as the old saying goes, when those appetites are unhealthy, "Garbage in, garbage out." Lust of the flesh refers to unhealthy relationships, and it doesn't necessarily mean romantic or sexual, though those certainly apply. It means pursuing things that are shallow in substance. The pursuit of people to feed our egos, who we can take from and not give back, and that includes those who pursue leadership positions in the church. Looking for what's in it for me or what can I get out of it instead of what can I give or what need can I fill for others instead of self. Lust of the eyes refers to the things we allow into the windows of our souls (Matthew 6:22). Matthews talks about what our pursuits are and if they are the shiny objects of the world and the sole focus of our passions is to attain those shiny objects, then the eye is diseased and better to have it removed than to go through life blinded by misguided passions. On the other hand, if our passionate pursuits are honorable and pleasing to God then the eye is healthy and vibrant. The eye was one of the areas that ultimately contributed to the downfall of Adam and Eve in Genesis. They were instructed to not eat from a certain tree, but "the woman saw that the tree was good for food, that it was pleasant to the eyes, and a tree desirable to make one wise, she took of its fruit and ate" (Genesis 3:6). Pleasure, desire, and lust are all fed through the eye and dictates what passions we will pursue desire is another form of the word "Appetite" in Greek.

Then there's the pride of life is the ill-fated pursuit of money, power, and prestige. It is the arrogance that my passions and pursuits are not in control, I am. It is the assumption that nothing, not even the devil, can control me, I am the captain of this ship. This person's passions are so misguided that they are willing to step on and over and to hurt anyone in their pursuit, including those closest to them, to get to the top of the mountain. The problem with that and almost always the case is that the higher you climb the greater the fall, and those same people that you stepped over and hurt on the way up you pass on the way down. It is why many celebrities struggle with depression and even commit suicide because that pursuit never ends, they reach one level and discover that it isn't enough. Pride is what drove Satan from heaven and according to the Bible, can drive us away as well, "Pride goes before destruction, And a haughty spirit before a fall" (Proverbs 16:18). This type of appetite is never nor can never be satisfied according to Ecclesiastes 6:7 and Isaiah 56:11. D. L. Moody may have said it best, "If we are full of pride and conceit and ambition and self-seeking and pleasure and the world, there is no room for the Spirit of God, and I believe many a man is praying to God to fill him when he is full already with something else." Pride is a shallow pursuit filled with landmines that are only designed to destroy.

I once heard a story about how our lives are likened to a house and we choose which areas of our lives we allow Jesus to come in and restore. Well one of those areas as the story is told, is our kitchen (our appetites). When we feed on junk foods such as cakes, candies, ice cream, and fried foods, they satisfy the short-term, but eventually, our overindulgence on those things produce all kinds of stomach issues, a tummy ache. However, when we allow the Lord into our kitchen, He prepares a nourishing and satisfying meal that is long-lasting, eternally. Again, our passionate pursuits can be satisfying short-term which leads to heartache and headache, or long-term which may encounter some turbulence, but ultimately will lead to health, mind, body, and spirit, and will lead to life eternal. The question then becomes what are our passions and how are they beneficial to not only me but to others? I know nurses who are passionate about helping the sick and hurting. They would do what they do day in and day out without pay because of the pleasure they receive from helping others despite occasional tragedies in their field. However, I also know nurses whose only passion is the paycheck. They come to work, they do their jobs, and most are very good at it, but they are not the most pleasant people toward those they are charged with caring for. Years ago, I had the thought of going to nursing school and sought the advice of a veteran peds RN who is also a friend, and what she told me initially shocked me. She said, "Do not do it if your only reason for doing so is the money, because you will be miserable no matter how much you make." And you know what? She was right. You must be passionate about what you do, but for the right reasons, and money, power, prestige, recognition is not even on the list. Do you want recognition? Passionately pursue the things of God and He will recognize you without you having to even ask for it. Whatever we feed on is what we crave, is what becomes our appetite. Solomon, in the passage at the beginning of this chapter, said if we are given over to self-defeating, self-destructive appetites, then you are taking a knife to your throat, and will ultimately be your undoing, and that's not God's best for you. Feed on those things which nourish and not destroy.

"Is it not the great end of religion, and, in particular, the glory of Christianity, to extinguish the malignant passions; to curb the violence, to control the appetites, and to

*smooth the asperities of man; to make us
compassionate and kind, and forgiving one
to another; to make us good husbands, good
fathers, good friends; and to render us active
and useful in the discharge of the relative
social and civil duties?"* William Wilberforce

Chapter II:

Strongholds

*"If you want to identify the hidden
strongholds in your life, you need only
survey the attitudes in your heart. Every
area in your thinking that glistens with hope
in God is an area which is being liberated by
Christ. But any system of thinking that does
not have hope, which feels hopeless, is a
stronghold which must be pulled down."*
Francis Frangipane

2 Corinthians 10:4-5, "For the weapons of our
warfare are not carnal but mighty in God for pulling
down strongholds, 5 casting down arguments and
every high thing that exalts itself against the
knowledge of God, bringing every thought into
captivity to the obedience of Christ" Strongholds in
many instances throughout Scripture is a good thing
because it represents security and safety. In Psalm
18:1-2 David refers to the Lord as his stronghold and
refuge and the minor prophet Nahum in 1:7 says that
the Lord is a stronghold to all who trust Him in times
of struggle. But then some strongholds give a false

sense of security and it is these that Paul has in mind. The word "Stronghold" translated from Greek, means any wrong thoughts, arguments, opinions, and opposition to the true knowledge nature of God. Things such as pride, selfishness, unforgiveness, and fear are all in opposition to the nature of God and His thoughts toward us and are ultimately a state of carnal thinking that will eventually lead to our destruction. Paul says that this mindset, this way of thinking cannot be fought with carnal weapons of war because their origin, while dripping with carnality, was introduced from a spiritual source, Satan and he uses certain things in our lives that are damaging as building blocks in the construction of those strongholds that not only not secure us, but actually make us prisoners in our minds. What are some of those things that he uses to begin to mix and mold those building blocks that imprison us?

Past hurts are one of the materials that get used to beginning to the process of enclosing us in this false sense of security. I remember hearing a story of a Missionary from Africa who was abused as a child by his stepfather. He noticed that the more he cried the more severe the beatings became, so he vowed to never cry again, to never show emotion because he viewed it as a sign of weakness. As a result, he created this false sense of strength by allowing anger to be the only emotion that could be displayed as it suggested toughness and authority. We previously discussed how damaging suppressing emotions can be and it unfortunate that many individuals undertake the same mentality because of past wounds like this gentleman from Africa. The good news is that this individual had an amazing encounter with Jesus that radically tore down those strongholds that kept him imprisoned for decades and transformed him into a mighty warrior for God. As he finished telling his story he said he discovered that openly displaying tears was not a sign of weakness but was, in fact, an opportunity to purge bad emotions and experiences to move forward.

Lies are another tactic that the enemy likes to use in abundance. He is referred to as the father of lies (John 8:44). He lied in the garden in telling Adam and Eve that they could be like God and he is still telling lies today. Even what is deemed as "Little white lies" can lead to a false sense of security. One of the "Little white lies" that has been displayed for all the world to see is on the T.V. shows American Idol. We all have seen the train wreckage from the auditions. Does anyone remember William Hung? And there have been plenty of other people whose family and friends convinced them that they can sing only to allow them to be made a mockery of at the expense of our entertainment. Now while this is a seemingly small issue, imagine the damage that can be inflicted on someone who goes through life thinking some lies that those closest to them have told them because we live in such a politically correct culture that honesty is viewed as a detriment. Lies feed us with this false sense of importance, worthiness, and security and is the primary weapon of war that the enemy uses.

Winston Churchill stated, "In wartime, truth is so precious that she should always be attended by a bodyguard of lies." We are in a spiritual battle Paul stated as much and trying to combat them with wrong thinking and motives will never gain us the victory.

Again, while we recognize that some strongholds are good and safe, there are others as Paul highlights, that produce wrong thinking which leads to wrongdoing because of a false sense of safety and ultimately imprisons us in our minds. Jesus indeed is a stronghold and refuge for those who put their trust in Him, but He must first begin to tear down those strongholds of offense and opposition to the things of God before He can reconstruct a fortress that is firm and strong. Those instruments used for the deconstruction are His Word, prayer, and the power of the Holy Spirit which is accessible to all who call on the name of the Lord.

> *"Where does your security lie? Is God your refuge, your hiding place, your stronghold, your shepherd, your counselor, your friend, your redeemer, your savior, your guide? If He is, you don't need to search any further for security."* Elisabeth Elliot

Pride

"No one enjoys feeling weak, whether it is emotionally, spiritually or physically. There is something within the human spirit that wants to resist the thought of weakness. Many times, this is nothing more than our human pride at work. Just as weakness carries a great potential for strength, pride carries an equally great potential for defeat."
Charles Stanley

1 Peter 5:5, "Likewise you younger people, submit yourselves to your elders. Yes, all of you be submissive to one another, and be clothed with humility, for "God resists the proud, But gives grace to the humble." I remember attending a men's conference up in the mountains with a small group of men from my church. There would be 200-300 men from several churches, with several speakers sharing stories of failures, struggles, and victories. Stories meant to encourage and inspire other men to be humble and trust in the Lord, and some of the stories shared were truly humbling, to say the least. However, the following story, of which I do not have permission to give names and give specific detail out of respect for

the individual, demonstrated anything but humility, and quite a few of the men in attendance took notice. It was a morning session and the speaker began very well by giving honor to God and thanking the men in attendance. Then it began. This individual began to truly boast about the insurance policy they had on their tongue, for you see this person was a taster for a large, well-known company, and his tongue was very special as they would repeatedly indicate. Also, this person bragged about how they single-handedly discovered a new flavor of the company's product and was solely responsible for procuring all the necessary ingredients to launch this new line of product. Furthermore, this individual had been invited to many Christian conferences, so it wasn't like maybe they were just nervous and innocently forgot to mention God. Well, let me just say that aside from the introduction, God was never again mentioned in their hour or so session, let alone given honor and praise for the gift that this individual had. One of the men that I sat with leaned over to me and said, "I thought they were going to talk about what God did for them?" Pride goes before destruction (Proverbs 16:18).

The word "Proud" is mentioned 47 times in the NKJV of the Bible, while "Pride" occurs 51 times, and means showing one's self above others, overtopping, conspicuous above others, pre-eminent. Pride was the reason Satan was cast from heaven (Isaiah 14:12-14) and was one of the original sins committed in the garden and pride continues to be an issue today. We live in a society that promotes self; self-confidence, self-reliant, self-sufficient, we have even corrupted a symbol of God's covenant with mankind (Genesis 9:13-16) and call it pride. Believe when I say that pride is a destroyer. It destroys relationships with family and friends, finances, eventually yourself because of the inability to recognize that nobody succeeds on their own, and in the grand scheme of things, no one succeeds without the Lord's blessings and favor. According to the word destruction from the Hebrew, it means breaking, fracture, crushing, breach, crash, and ultimate ruin. Pride is the poison of the soul and is one of the six things that the Lord hates, the strongest word for hate used in the Hebrew language, according to Proverbs 16:5. And as previously mentioned, it was the precursor to all sin because it was the very thing that causes the father of sin to be thrown out of heaven.

Pride is a destroyer because it leads to things such as conceit, strife, and counterfeits. Pride and conceit go hand in hand because pride insists on the fact that the person has accomplished their success all by themselves and therefore have no need for anyone. As a result of conceit, the prideful individual push people away and thereby begin to neglect and even destroy relationships. Strife's role in the prideful is the desire to always be first, second place will never be enough. To this person, even things that should be for entertainment such as bowling or board games become a competition for them, striving to be number one. Remember what the Bible says about those who insist on being first. On the very night that the Lord would be betrayed and led off to His eventual execution, the disciples began to argue over who would be the greatest in heaven at the Lord's supper (Luke 22:24). The Word says that there was a great dispute and the word used for a dispute in the Greek is the word strife. And according to Proverbs 6:19, one of the other things that the Lord hates in addition to pride is a person causes discord or strife between people. Now I can only imagine that the Lord was like "Really guys? C'mon." However, Jesus simply used this opportunity to teach them what is expected of a follower of His and who was the model for that lifestyle. Luke 25-27 says, "And He said to them, "The kings of the Gentiles exercise lordship over them, and those who exercise authority over them are called 'benefactors.' But not so among you; on the contrary, he who is greatest among you, let him be as the younger, and he who governs as he who serves. For who is greater, he who sits at the table, or he who serves? Is it not he who sits at the table? Yet I am among you as the One who serves."

People who are conceited and always striving because of pride eventually become counterfeits. They are counterfeits because when they do not reach the intended successes that they are striving for, and is almost always the case, they will become motivated to put on an act for a show to disguise the fact that they have had failures. And because their whole persona is so caught up in being number one and being the best, that failure or accepting less would never do, as a result, they must put on airs to portray something that they are not. Ultimately, these individuals become disingenuous, insincere, unreliable. Eventually, prideful people become untrustworthy because others view them as less than honest and shallow. Relationships are bonded on the idea that you can trust the other person and that is not in that relationship just for themselves, and when trust is violated it becomes very difficult to restore. As a result, prideful people are often isolated even in a crowd because people see through the facade and want nothing to do with them. Pride is a destroyer because it elevates a person above even the Lord Himself, and trust me when I tell you, He is not sharing His throne or title with anyone. Finally, pride is a destroyer because it leads to rejecting the help of others, causes us to become blind to the fact that we are prideful, eventually to a selfish and self-serving mentality which will be covered in the next chapter, and it is no wonder that John R. W. Stott said, "Pride is your greatest enemy, humility is your greatest friend." According to the passage in this chapter, God gives grace to the humble. Grace, unmerited and undeserved favor from all that heaven holds becomes accessible to the humble. The idea that humility is a weakness is a myth. It is recognizing that there are some things that I simply am unable to do on my own, that there are others who are capable of offering help and vice versa if we humble ourselves. It is recognizing that NO ONE is better than the next and that Jesus died for the entire world, not just a select few choice individuals. But be warned, false humility which is self-defeating and people-pleasing because it is looking for attention and recognition which is pride in disguise.

> "The Christian Gospel is that I am so flawed that Jesus had to die for me, yet I am so loved and valued that Jesus was glad to die for me. This leads to deep humility and deep confidence at the same time. It undermines both swaggering and sniveling. I cannot feel superior to anyone, and yet I have nothing to prove to anyone. I do not think more of myself nor less of myself. Instead, I think of myself less." Timothy Keller

Selfishness

"The poison of selfishness destroys the world." Catherine of Siena

Philippians 2:3 says, "Let nothing be done through selfish ambition or conceit, but in lowliness of mind let each esteem others better than himself." You would be surprised to discover that the word "Selfish" does not appear in the original languages (Greek, Aramaic, Hebrew) of the Bible. Instead, the word that is translated into English as selfish is the word "Strife," which appears 31 times in the NKJV of the Bible and means; a desire to put one's self forward, a partisan and fractious spirit. There are four very important issues standing out in this passage that is worth mentioning; two negatives; selfish ambition and conceit, two positives; lowliness of mind and esteem others better or higher than self. Let us unpack each of these one at a time and the first is selfish ambition.

Ambition by itself is not the issue. I think we can agree that everyone has some type of ambition. An ambition to get healthier, to attain a higher degree, start a family, and grow in a closer relationship with the Lord, all of which are commendable. When someone has healthy ambitions, they are determined to work hard to achieve their goals, understanding that nothing worth having comes apart from commitment and hard work. When the decision was made for me to return to school after 30 years removed from a classroom, I had one objective in mind, work hard to attain my degree and do it above the board. However, the issue occurs when those ambitions come with the high price of compromising core values and integrity or at the expense of another by devaluing or taking advantage of people to achieve a specific goal. Individuals who achieve success at the expense of others are manipulative and deceitful. As a result, these individuals are typically shallow in character and are only surrounded by people who feed into their ego. These people only want to be the center of attention and will resort to mocking the struggles and failures of others to gain attention and make themselves feel better about themselves. Those who are driven by selfish pursuits do so by taking advantage of others and have no concern with seeing others hurt if it will mean their success. For example, throughout 2 Samuel we read about how Absalom lied, cheated, and divided his family in his pursuit to become king of Israel. People and relationships are devalued if the self-driven individual is not the most important member of that relationship. Self-ambitious individuals are full of themselves, typically narcissistic, and have an elevated of who they are and their abilities, conceited.

Conceit or vainglory as the Word refers to and pride, one could say, are kissing cousins, and the wisest individual in the Bible, Solomon, wrote throughout Ecclesiastes and Proverbs about the dangers and failing of thinking more of oneself than you ought to think. thinking to. Those who are conceited have put a high value on their way of thinking and doing and because of this are very on teachable. Solomon highlights that in Provers 26:12, "Do you see a man wise in his own eyes? There is more hope for a fool than for him." These are the type to never accept the fact that they are wrong sometimes even when it is obvious that they are. I remember in one of my first classes back in school there was this one student that just knew he was the next scholar, that he even thought he was smarter than the professor of the class who had 20 plus years' experience as an educator and the Graduate level degree to go with it. And yet with all of this, that student would frequently debate this professor on various topics in class even though they were misinformed. But in their mind, because of conceit, you couldn't tell this individual anything because being wrong sometimes was never a consideration for them. That's why 1 Corinthians 1:27 says, "But God has chosen the foolish things of the world to put to shame the wise, and God has chosen the weak things of the world to put to shame the things which are mighty," because those who are full of themselves cannot be full of the things of God. For this reason, the self-ambitious and conceited need to first be humbled before God can use them. However, with humility comes lowliness of mind.

From the Greek, lowliness of mind means a deep sense of one's (moral) littleness. In other words, it is understanding that we are need of a Savior because we recognize that we all suffer from some degree of selfishness and self-centeredness. It is also an acute awareness of our littleness in the grand scheme of the universe and how grand and awe-inspiring the Creator of that universe is. I remember the moment that I realized just how insignificant I am in the grand scheme of things, which was a truly humbling moment. My wife and I chartered a boat from Newport to Catalina Island for a little mini vacation. The boat cruise was nice, the weather was very agreeable, and we were on our way. However, there came a point in our trip where you could no longer see Newport and Catalina had yet to come into view, and all there was before us the vastness of the Pacific Ocean. I distinctly remember experiencing this overwhelming awareness of how truly small I was against the backdrop of this ocean. But you what is even more humbling than that, realizing that just because we are barely specks in this vast universe, God thinks tremendously about us. I think David said it best in Psalm 8:3-5, "When I consider Your heavens, the work of Your fingers, The moon, and the stars, which You have ordained, What is man that You are mindful of him, And the son of man that You visit[a] him? For You have made him a little lower than the angels, And You have crowned him with glory and honor." When we consider this, it should drive us to humility and as a result, it becomes very easy to consider others above us.

   The King of the universe said He came to serve and not be served (Matthew 20:28) as a template for His followers to replicate and this is not negotiable. We must get to a point, myself included, of seeing people as Jesus saw them, even the ones who reject Him. Esteeming others above self is not a self-demoting or self-defeating premise. It is recognizing that as I have been given gifts and blessings, they were not given to be to horde but to continue the flow of God's goodness toward humanity. It is through encouraging and facilitating other people's growth that we begin to grow, not through self-promotion and selfish pursuits. Paul was highlighting the culture of the time that looked at humility as a weakness to be exploited and is the culture of our time as well. And just a Jesus was a true rebel and revolutionary in terms of disrupting destructive cultures, we are called to do the same as we become more Christ-like. That was the thing that attracted people to Jesus was His counter-culture lifestyle and message, and He commissioned us to do the same, John 14:12, "Most assuredly, I say to you, he who believes in Me, the works that I do he will do also; and greater works than these he will do, because I go to My Father," and that work is selfless.

   "Selfishness is the controlling force of sinful living. It is this motive which pulsates

through the natural mind, emotions and will
- self-pleasing, self-serving, living for self."
Walter J. Chantry

Unforgiveness

"Forgiveness is the key that unlocks the door of resentment and the handcuffs of hatred. It is a power that breaks the chains of bitterness and the shackles of selfishness."
Corrie Ten Boom

Mark 11:25-26, "And whenever you stand praying, if you have anything against anyone, forgive him, that your Father in heaven may also forgive you your trespasses. But if you do not forgive, neither will your Father in heaven forgive your trespasses." There are a variety of implications from the original language (Greek) in the word "forgive," but the two that I find intriguing are "to leave to go to another place" and "to go away leaving something behind." That is what Jesus is highlighting here, when we are in prayer or corporately worshipping and unforgiveness is brought to remembrance, leave where you are at and go make things right if we want to experience deeper intimacy in worship and receive greater blessings that naturally follow. If when you are offering up your prayers for blessings, provisions, protection, and guidance, we are also likely to remember those who have wronged us in the past, and therefore the Lord is saying "Before I can bless, heal, or guide in the present or future, I need you to release the past." Essentially, we should stop right there and go release the burden of unforgiveness before we can expect God's intervention in our lives. And as a reminder and incentive, Remember the reason that Jesus came to earth, to do the Father's will in dealing with our sins justly that He may forgive our sins righteously.

The idea is to leave or abandon that which keeps us anchored in the past, stuck in the present and prevents us from moving forward into something better. Unforgiveness keeps us stuck in the mire of past hurts and past struggles and prevents us from moving into new opportunities for healing and blessing. I remember on my first mission trip to Nicaragua and listening to one of our leaders talk about how some healings are hindered by retaining unforgiveness, and such would be the case on the last crusade in Nicaragua. This would be our largest crusade in terms of those who would attend and the volume of ministering to the needs of those in attendance, roughly 1,200-1,500 people not counting the vendors that came out to sell their wares. Early on during the event, I met this vendor who happened to know several of the host church's leadership and through my interpreter, we had a brief conversation just about the event itself. However, toward the end where an invitation was offered to come forward for anyone that wanted prayer for salvation, healing, and deliverance. To my surprise, this vendor came forward. After a few probing questions, I would discover through my interpreter that this person had been hurt and discarded by their family and had been holding onto that for decades. When we began to pray, one of the things that needed to take place was to leave the past in the past to move into newness of life and healing (forgiveness). Once this was able to take place, this individual began to weep like a child and release all that pain and replace it with peace. They were able to leave pain and anguish in the past and move into a place of blessing and freedom.

What forgiving does is it frees us from the past and from people which then allows us to move into newness of life. I remember hearing about a woman who had been abused by a trusted family member as a child and for over 30 years, had been carrying around this shame, hurt, and as a result, unforgiveness. Now I won't try to devalue or diminish the tragedy of any type of abuse, it is horrible and tragic for the abused. However, I will say that when we refuse to forgive as difficult as it might be, we are continuing to allow the abuser to wield power over us. Foreverness does not require an apology from the one who hurt us and violated our trust, but what it does do is let them know what the did, as unacceptable as it was, will no longer keep us stuck in the past. It allows us to take back that part of our lives and move forward into healing, blessing, and liberty. Unfortunately, this life will have its moments of difficulties, which include heartache and disappointment from those who we have allowed into our inner circle. Jesus said as much, "In the world, you will have tribulation; but be of good cheer, I have overcome the world" (John 16:33). And while He was speaking broadly, I cannot imagine that He didn't include betrayal by those to whom we have put our trust and confidence. The problem is that life does not have a rewind button and therefore makes it nearly impossible to go back and undo what has been done. However, what we can do is forgive the past offense and move forward regardless if the one who has wronged us acknowledges the offense or apologizes.

I think I was around 5 years old that I first recall the physical abuse that I suffered at the hands of a stepbrother. Made to ingest things that are not intended to be ingested, forced to drink mass amounts of water to force vomiting and then made to sleep in it, and lost both my front teeth at his hands. To say that our home was a house of horror would be a slight understatement. Eventually, we would be forced from this home and went on with our lives. Now time is a funny thing, unknown to us, it passes by so quickly and 40 years removed from that period of my life is no longer a thought, nor have I had contact with that individual in 40 years. One morning I returned home from our regular men's fellowship to discover I had a message from that individual on my phone with this long sincere message of ownership and remorse. He went on to say that he would completely understand if I did not respond, he would expect nothing less but just wanted to express his deepest apology and asked for forgiveness. Wow! I had not thought about this period of my life for 40 years and now this flood of memories and emotions came to the forefront. What could I do? I mean naturally speaking, I had the right to withhold forgiveness and retain that anger and hurt. However, I am now in ministry and preach on forgiveness and moving forward, and that is what I did, I forgave him. I responded to his message after processing it and my emotions and explained to him that I had not thought about him or that time in my life, and furthermore, was in the business of forgiveness. I cannot say that the heavens opened, and doves filled the air, but what I can say is that there was the kind of peace that I experienced. And though the pain from the past, which had been stowed away, unknown to me had to be addressed and let go of. Past hurts and offenses are difficult to deal with let alone forgiven, but the Lord says it must be that way to receive the full forgiveness of the Father. The expression goes "Let go and let God," and as simple as that sounds, it is true. God must be the one to heal us from past pain, but He cannot do so until we release it.

> *"Unforgiveness is a prison. It slams the door on new beginnings and entrenches you in your present pain. It chains the heart and stops it from beating. It suffocates joy and paralyzes your ability to move on. Unforgiveness is the cancer of the soul. It slowly eats away the marrow of your existence and impairs your judgment, your personality and your ability to love again."*
> Michelle McKinney Hammond

Fear

"Fear is born of Satan, and if we would only take time to think a moment we would see that everything Satan says is founded upon a falsehood." A. B. Simpson

1 John 4:18 "There is no fear in love [dread does not exist], but full-grown (complete, perfect) love turns fear out of doors and expels every trace of terror! For fear brings with it the thought of punishment, and [so] he who is afraid has not reached the full maturity of love [is not yet grown into love's complete perfection]." Fear in its natural state is an appropriate emotion or reaction because it is a type of warning sign against potential danger. Furthermore, the word "fear" is mentioned 124 times in the Bible, which is a benefit for those who have a healthy fear and reverence of the Lord. For example, Psalm 25:14 says, "The secret of the Lord is with those who fear Him, And He will show them His covenant." And Proverbs 9:10 says, "The fear of the Lord is the beginning of wisdom, And the knowledge of the Holy One is understanding." So, fear of the Lord produces the benefit of intimacy, counsel, and godly wisdom just to name a few. However, the fear that the Apostle

John is talking about here is one of dread, terror, and panic. It is where we get the word "phobia," which is an irrational fear that cripples millions of people daily. This fear is direct opposition to the perfect love of God, you cannot have one while being consumed by the other.

Like unforgiveness, fear can inhibit the blessings of the Lord and imprison us in our minds, and in some cases can paralyze us. Some of the things that fear can do to us physically are incredibly dangerous, such as lower our immune system, cardiovascular digestive damage. Fear can hinder or inhibit our long-term memory, inhibit our ability to regulate rational fear from irrational, which ultimately hinders our ability to regulate our emotions. Finally, long-term, unresolved fears can begin to cause us to develop other mental health issues such as depression, anxiety, and PTSD, none of which are symbolic of the natural and healthy fear nor of the perfect love of God actively at work in us, and John is saying violates God's promise perfect peace to us. Phobos or phobia in one of the most common forms of mental illness in America today. Approximately 10% of Americans suffer some type of phobia, 7% of which are social phobias according to The National Institute of Mental Health. Social phobias, now referred to as social anxiety disorder, include anything having to do with engaging with society and can be as severe as refusing to leave the house at all. It is brought on by the fear of being embarrassed or scrutinized by the public. Essentially, this type of fear that John is talking about, one of dread, panic, and doom, is so preoccupied with external and temporal things that these individuals are unable to see the spiritual things of God.

Fear contrasts with the boldness of the Lord that we are called to walk in because of the perfect love of God infused into our spirits. It is an internal work that displays the transformed life that has been imparted and that is not afraid to speak about our faith in the Lord openly. The word used in 1 John 4:18 for perfect means wanting nothing necessary to completeness, finished as in Jesus' victory cry on the cross in John 19:30 which a variation of the Greek word "teleios," or "perfect." Jesus' perfect love displayed in crimson on a tree over 2,00 years ago made it possible for us not to dread the righteous judgment of God, and to boldly display that grace in mercy in our actions and our speech regardless of what others think or feel. And while we are told not to purposely offend people, which means that we do NOT get to pass judgment upon those outside the Church family (1 Corinthians 5). We do, however, with grace and the motivation to bring healing and awareness of true worth (Colossians 4:6), challenge thought and action. We must remember that the author of fear has also blinded the eyes who oppose the truth and only through perfect love and truth can we begin to take those blinders off, which means that there can be no fear in us about this newfound perfect love that has been given. Jack Hayford stated, "How would you treat a friend who lied to you as much as your fears do?" The answer is that we would get rid of them quickly, and perfect love does that for us if we will get out of the way and let the Lord do the heavy lifting for us. Unfortunately, like Abraham, we think we can take matters into our own hands to help God out, the results are never good.

Where perfect love is not allowed to take root and grow, like an unwanted weed on the lawn, dread and panic begin to grow which becomes the irrational fear and concerned about what others might think or say about us. Bill Johnson stated in his book "When Heaven Invades Earth," "If you live off a man's compliments, you'll die from his criticism." The fact of the matter is many of us, including myself, if we are being honest tend to shrink when the opportunity arises for us to speak about our faith out of fear of offending. Unfortunately, the gospel is offensive because while it offers forgiveness of sin for all, it is also intolerant of sin which is an offense to God. to those who either do not see that their lifestyle of selfish pursuits and self-serving mindsets are offensive to God or those individuals who believe in God, read their Word, attend Church, but you would never know in public that they are believers of Christ because they blend in with the world. These are referred to as "closet" Christians, afraid to come out of the closet for fear of rejection, embarrassment, and abandonment by those closest to them, which is an irrational fear and is in direct contradiction to the perfect love of God. We cannot afford to allow external factors to govern what rightfully belongs to God internally by our confession of Jesus as our Savior. We must be willing to accept that there will be those who reject our new life and will mock us and leave us. Fear in its pure state can be helpful, but when it is misplaced or irrational then it can be deadly. Matthew 10:28 says, "And do not fear those who kill the body but cannot kill the soul. But rather fear Him who can destroy both soul and body in hell." The question we need to be asking ourselves is who are we more worried over offending, God or people? The answer has eternal consequences. Do we choose to bask in the perfect love of God, or do we wallow in the mire and despair of irrational fear, dread, and doom? A friend of mine in India has a young son, Aaron Moktan, offered such profound wisdom in the following statement, "There are 3 Cs in life, Choice, chance, and change. We have to choose to take a chance if we want anything to change in our lives," so choose wisely.

> *"God incarnate is the end of fear; and the heart that realizes that, realizes that he is in the midst, that takes heed to the assurance of his loving presence, will be quiet in the midst of alarm."* F. B. Meyer

Chapter III:

Understanding

"The first source of sin is error in the understanding, which is the natural guide and counselor of the will. Consequently, the chief endeavor of the devil is to darken the understanding, and thus draw the will into the same error. Thus he clothes evil with the appearance of good, and presents vice under the mask of virtue, that we may regard it as a counsel of reason rather than a temptation of the enemy." Louis of Granada

Proverbs 3:5-6 says, "Trust in the Lord with all your heart, And lean not on your understanding; In all your ways acknowledge Him, And He shall direct your paths." Solomon is teaching his son, I think, highlighted four areas worth noting in these two verses; Trust, lean, our understanding, and acknowledge. I think it is important to address each one of these independently to catch the depth of these words. Trust is the first on the list. Trust is a very valuable and yet fragile thing because it involves investing a part of ourselves, namely our heart, to something and someone. The issue is the thing or person in which we commit our trust to will either elevate us or sink us, because that is where we have placed the most value. Jesus said in Matthew 6:21, "For where your treasure is, there your heart will be also." Wherever we have committed our hearts to trust, there our treasure will be. The issue is that it is often misplaced toward wealth, power, recognition, and ill-advised relationships. The results often cost us more than we are prepared to pay, such as careers, finances, and important relationships because we have elevated other things above what is important by allowing our hearts to trust in meaningless pursuits. Solomon is saying, "Do not do that. Stop relying on things that are shallow or worthless. Our trust should belong to the Lord and Him alone, and if we will trust Him then everything will fall into place."

Which brings us to leaning. The Hebrew definition of the word means to use something or someone we rely on as support. Support can be a good thing, especially if you are struggling with something. Having someone to talk to or to lean on is vitally important. In Exodus 17, when Israel went up against the Amalekites, it was going to take a praying Moses and the mighty hand of God to achieve the victory. Often that is how victory is won, by unceasing prayer. Unfortunately, Moses began to get weary and if it were not for the ability to lean on Aaron and Hur, who knows how the battle would have come out. However, most of the time we lean on our finances, jobs, and substances for support in times of difficulties. Again, the results are often tragic because we are leaning on the wrong thing. Isaiah 31:1 says. "Woe to those who go down to Egypt for help, And rely on horses, Who trust in chariots because they are many, And in horsemen because they are very strong, But who do not look to the Holy One of Israel, Nor seek the Lord!" Because all of those things, despite our understanding of those things, are unreliable compared to the surety of the Lord.

One of the other things we rely on just a bit too much is our intellect. I have said it before, there are roughly 18 inches between heaven and hell. Proverbs 26:4 says, "Do not answer a fool according to his folly, Lest you also be like him." Why? Because they can never be reasoned with, they must be humbled by the Lord. The Law of the Lord has to be used as a pickax, breaking up the hardened soil of the heart before the pure seed of the Word can be planted in hopes of establishing deep roots. That is why Paul said in Galatians 3:24, that the Law was a schoolmaster (King James version), instructing us of our inability to keep our moral standing with the Lord in our understanding. When we infuse our intellect into the things of God, they become subjective versus objective, meaning that God's standards are flexible according to each person's understanding of them which is a destructive path to travel. Leaning on our understanding is limited by design and this was first evident in the Garden of Eden when Adam and Eve were instructed not to eat from Tree of the Knowledge of Good and Evil. God didn't put limits to control us but to preserve us from the temptations of the world, but the serpent had other ideas. As a result of irrational thinking brought about by the ability of Satan to manipulate rational thought, Adam and Eve defied God and paid the price for it. Our reasoning is prone to manipulation and therefore cannot be fully trusted, which is why we need evidence-based logic and rational to make an informed decision. However, when we lean on God's omnipotent and eternal understanding, we can trust that He will guide our paths for His name's sake.

Which brings us to the final point, simply acknowledge all that is the goodness and glory of the Lord. Our ability to cite passages of the Bible, to when souls to the Kingdom, pray for the sick and see them recovered, and visit the widows and orphans are meaningless unless we acknowledge that if were not for the Lord these things would be meaningless. Do not misunderstand, God is not some deity saying, "Pay attention to me." But He is worthy of all the praise and adoration for who He is and what He has done for us. The Father sent His Son to pay our death penalty, for that He is deserving of acknowledgment. He has imparted to us His Spirit to help us in this life, for that He is worthy to be acknowledged. Finally, when we do acknowledge Him, He reveals to us our true identity as sons and daughters of the Most High God. That means the titles that the world, the flesh, and the Devil himself try to ascribe to us no longer have value or importance. Things like self-doubt, guilt, shame, and condemnation are no longer in our vocabulary, only righteousness, peace, and salvation remain. When we trust in Him, rely on Him, acknowledge Him, God lays out our path to eternity and ensures that as long as we stay the course, He will see to it that we finish the journey which ends when we come face to face with our Savior, because He is directing us by His gentle Spirit.

"Real satisfaction comes not in understanding God's motives, but in understanding His character, in trusting in His promises, and in leaning on Him and resting in Him as the Sovereign who knows what He is doing and does all things well." Joni Eareckson Tada

Doubt

"Doubt discovers difficulties which it never solves; it creates hesitancy, despondency, despair. Its progress is the decay of comfort, the death of peace. "Believe!" is the word which speaks life into a man, but doubt nails down his coffin." Charles Spurgeon

James 1:5-8 says, "If any of you lacks wisdom, let him ask of God, who gives to all liberally and without reproach, and it will be given to him. But let him ask in faith, with no doubting, for he who doubts is like a wave of the sea driven and tossed by the wind. For let, not that man suppose that he will receive anything from the Lord; he is a double-minded man, unstable in all his ways." The word used for "doubting," from the Greek, is mentioned 24 times in 18 verses in the NKJV and is the word waver. The word "waver" essentially means to hesitate, become indecisive, and to dispute against self. In the context of the passage in James, it is doubting your God-given abilities, and in so doing, doubting God. To allow doubt to take root in our hearts and mind is to say that the God of the universe, who has imparted His Spirit into us, is not able to do what He says He can do or is untrue to His

Word. Doubt is an enemy of faith. For example, James said, "If any of you lacks wisdom, let him ask of God, who gives to all liberally and without reproach." That word "reproach" means without regret of bestowing His gifts to us, and James continues by saying "it will be given to him.," If we ask in faith, it is saying that we believe God has, in the past and will do so again in the present. "But let him ask in faith, with no doubting," for in doubting we are relying on unstable ground to hold us up instead of the stable Word of God, the Bible instructs against that, "Let us hold fast the confession of our hope without wavering, for He who promised is faithful" (Hebrews 10:23). What is interesting about that passage is that just before v.23 it says that we have now been given access to the very throne room of God through Jesus and are invited to come with full assurance (v.22), meaning lacking any doubt. And right after, it says that we must live by faith (v.38) and therefore not to discard our enduring hope (v.35).

Of course, I won't say that sometimes our faith gets beat up and hanging by a thread. I will just say that because we know God has a track record of coming through in times of need, that He will again, we just need to ask and believe. Think of that poor father in Mark 9 with the demon-possessed son that he brought to the Lord in his darkest time. He had enough faith to believe that God can and will deliver even in his weakness. Check out what he said, "Immediately the father of the child cried out and said with tears, "Lord, I believe; help my unbelief!" (v.24).

God blesses and imparts to us our identity and value, so why would He simply ignore us in our times of trial as is the context of James' instruction to the Church here. Doubt in the mind is a constant tug of war over believing and rejecting what God says He will do and who we are to Him, in Him, and through Him. Now if you are like me, you also struggle with getting out of your head when it comes to ignoring the voices that say "You are not good enough, smart enough, capable enough, or loved enough and therefore should just stop trying." That is the voice of the enemy trying to get you to buy into the mindset of the old nature that was truly corrupt and misguided. However, that was not our intended purpose of creation. God made us in His image, which means that we were destined for great things. He also breathed His breath of life into us, and the word used for breath there in Genesis 2 is the same word used for His Spirit. Therefore, not only were we made to reflect the image of perfection, but He imparted His Spirit to ensure that His image would not be altered, distorted, or changed. Unfortunately, that serpent of old deceived our first parents and thereby corrupted that which should have been pure and undefiled. Thus, doubt among other things, was birthed, and that same serpent of old is now trying to keep corruption alive, and the lie of doubting God and His impartations to us is one of his main tactics.

When I was pursuing my degree, I was surrounded by other students 20 years younger than me and continuing their education with no breaks in between compared to my 30-year absence from school. As a result, I was always challenged with the thought that I was not smart enough, capable enough, skilled enough, good enough to achieve my goal of acquiring this degree and therefore had no business being here. There were times that the doubt was so overwhelming that I was prepared to quit. In my mind, I was unstable and indecisive by all the negativity and doubt that I was consuming my thoughts. What's worse is I had been a follower of Jesus for several years at this point, been on numerous mission trips and seen the hand of God in action, led many to the Lord, and yet wavered in my God-given abilities. Fortunately, I have some well-grounded believers in the Lord who continued to encourage, instruct, and even offer a little kick in the rear to remind me that I have the mind of Christ (1 Corinthians 2:16) and that I could do anything I set my mind to do. As a result, I graduated with honors simply because I doubted my doubts and believed God for success. I think there is one purpose, among several, in Jesus going to the cross for us that is grossly undervalued and overlooked. While it is certainly true that He came to pay the penalty, we deserved for sin as justice had to be paid and righteousness restored, first and foremost (Romans 3:25, Hebrews 2:17, 1 John 2:2 and 4:10). However, Jesus also came to restore our rightful place in creation that was surrendered in the garden by our first parents. Our created value and purpose had been robbed. Jesus took back what once was (Romans 8:19-23, Galatians 4:4 and then returned it to us upon our confession of Jesus as our Savior and Redeemer. However, the one I like best is 2 Corinthians 5:17, "Therefore, if anyone is in Christ, he is a new creation; old things have passed away; behold, all things have become new." I like it because the word "new" has the idea of a package that has never been disturbed, torn, or destroyed. It is restored to its original state, which was our previous state through the events in Eden. How befitting it is in that the process of restoring that which was stolen in the garden of Eden, began in another garden, Gethsemane, and of this fact, there can be no doubting otherwise the enemy wins.

Finally, James says "If any of you lack, are found to be wanting, to be destitute... ask." Now here he is referring to wisdom, but Jesus repeatedly in one form or another stated that we should readily seek Him out for all that we need after all one of His names is the All-Sufficient One. I think we all agree that we have moments where we feel utterly empty and devoid of confidence and assurance that success is attainable. It has been said that it has been stated that we battle against three enemies; Satan, the world, and self. Of the three, I think we battle the most with self, though I think the other two play supporting roles feeding into our feeble minds that we are not smart enough, strong enough, or capable enough to accomplish our God-given purpose. James is saying in those moments of emptiness or lack, "take a timeout, seek the Lord, and ask Him for what you need at that moment." And the Father promises that He will supply all our needs according to His riches in Christ Jesus (Philippians

4:19) as all that we are is found in Jesus. The best part of this passage in James is that He will provide for need simply, sincerely, bountifully, and unconditionally. Why? Because that is who He is. However, when we ask if must be of singleness of heart, even in our weakness and doubt. It must be from a place of genuine brokenness and contrition that we seek freedom from the bondage of doubt, especially the doubting of our identity in Jesus. Remember the father from Mark 9, "I believe, but I need help with my doubts." Doubting is the enemy of faith. It is founded on lies that deny our created value, purpose, and ultimately it doubts that authority and sovereignty of God. Doubt your doubts, stop listening to the voices that say "you are not good enough," and start believing God when He says "You can do all things through Christ who strengthens you" (Philippians 4:13), and when the voices of the world, the flesh, or Satan rise up, just simply ask the God of abundance to increase faith and wisdom to combat those doubting voices.

"My child, don't be childish. But consider the child whose faith has not quite learned the definition of impossible. Have your questions. I'm not telling you to have blind faith. I'm telling you to consider the blind men who had faith and believed My Words before they were even able to see Me. Consider the birds that eat from My hand and do not fall from the sky without My consent so how much more will I love the

ones that I died for? Before you doubt Me, doubt your doubts. Doubt your doubts and you will see they are just as empty as the tomb that I walked from." Joseph Solomon

Guilt

"What I've seen is that everywhere, both Christians and non-Christians are held in bondage by guilt and condemnation. Satan is the accuser, and we don't want to stand in agreement with him. His desire is to take the world to hell with him." Robbie Dawkins

Romans 8:12-16 says, "Therefore, brethren, we are debtors—not to the flesh, to live according to the flesh. For if you live according to the flesh you will die; but if by the Spirit you put to death the deeds of the body, you will live. For as many as are led by the Spirit of God, these are sons of God. For you did not receive the spirit of bondage again to fear, but you received the Spirit of adoption by whom we cry out, "Abba, Father." The word "bondage," in the context of the period in which Paul writes, indicates one who is enslaved to a thing or object or person. In this case, Paul also includes the word debtor, thus suggesting that those who are in bondage, serve a specific master to whom they are in debt to until such a time that the debt is satisfied. Therefore, considering this passage, we were enslaved by sin and as a result, debtors to God for payment of sin. In other words, are involved in behavior in contradiction to the Law of God, made us guilty as charged by that same Law. For the Christian, according to the International Standard Bible Encyclopedia, the idea of guilt involves three elements: responsibility (cause, depending upon a man's real freedom), blameworthiness (depending upon a man's knowledge and purpose) and the obligation to make good through punishment or compensation (debt). In other words, in thinking of guilt we ask the questions of cause, motive, and consequence, the central idea being that of the personal blameworthiness of the sinner. All these elements keep us in bondage as debtors against God and humanity, the Law made it clear that because no one can fulfill the Law perfectly, will be deemed guilty and deserving of God's righteous judgment. So, let us unpack the three elements of guilt, the bondage that it creates, and the freedom we must now claim through Jesus' finished work on the cross of Calvary.

Responsibility or cause of guilt can be traced back to the very beginning, back to the Garden of Eden. God created man, gave him authority over God's creation, and simply asked of him one thing, "DO NOT eat of the tree of the knowledge of good and evil" (Genesis 2:17). Simple enough instructions, right? However, we know the rest of the story from Genesis 3, the serpent deceived Eve, Eve gave to Adam, and so here we are. But, aside from the blatant disregard for God's instructions, there was another sinful act on display that fateful day. No one took responsibility for their actions. Eve blamed the serpent, Adam blamed

Eve, but no one took responsibility for their actions, and that seems to be the story today. As someone who works in the field of psychology, and more specifically, in educating about addictions, I inform groups that the first step to any recovery is taking ownership or responsibility. Until a person takes responsibility, recovery is impossible. Therefore, the cause or responsibility for the guilt of sin is deferring or deflecting blame, the serpent did it, my wife made me do it, the boss made me mad, my peers pressured me into doing it. Whatever the excuse, as long as it is not my fault, and yet this is where the bondage of guilt begins to take root, weighing us down with the burden of poor choices and actions that are no judged by the high standards of God's Law, and thereby surrendering our freedom. The verdict, guilty as charged because we should have known better, which brings us to blameworthiness or knowledge and purpose.

Again, restating the origin of guilt, which was brought on by sinful acts, was in the garden. However, what was that act in question? Disobeying God's command to not eat from the tree of the knowledge of good and evil. In a quest for knowledge at the behest of the serpent provoking the interest and curiosity of Eve and purposeful pursuit, the deed was done. Listen to how the serpent framed the enticement, "For God knows that in the day you eat of it your eyes will be opened, and you will be like God, knowing good and evil" (Genesis 3:5). It was the false sense of knowing what God knows for becoming a god (little g) themselves, for the word "know" used in this passage has the idea of making oneself known. It is stating that I am my god by denying our Creator and promoting self which is exactly what the enemy wants you to do. Unfortunately, knowing isn't all that great, because knowledge doesn't equate to having the ability to do. For example, many wish that they knew the day that they would die because then they could prepare or go out with a blaze of glory only to discover that knowing only brings with it sadness and despair. And those who are determined to be their gods soon discover that knowing when they would die doesn't allow them to stop death from coming, having, therefore, wasted their purpose, are stuck with the guilt of rejecting God, and only have the self to blame. Knowledge is a good thing, but knowledge can produce pride and arrogance, and when that happens, the true knowledge which comes from fellowship with God vanishes away. According to research conducted in 2018 by Lifeway Research, Two-thirds (66 percent) of American young adults who attended a Protestant church regularly for at least a year as a teenager say they also dropped out for at least a year between the ages of 18 and 22. Part of that is parents teaching their kids about church routine instead of the Person and works of Jesus. However, as one who attending higher education as an older student, I saw firsthand how in many cases educators are force-feeding these young minds with knowledge that is hostile to the faith, and by oversaturating these minds that are still developing, they are able to influence, like the serpent, these young people into pursuing knowledge that in opposition to God. Now I am not saying that higher learning is a bad thing, far from it. I am just saying that the pursuit of knowledge can be dangerous if we are not careful about from which tree we partake because it just might put us in debt.

In thinking about debt, I think about people's frantic scramble at Christmas time looking for the perfect gift for a beloved or ensuring that the children have everything that they put on their Wishlist. Unfortunately, this is where many go into debt with their credit card companies and are left with trying to devise ways of repairing the damage left by overextending oneself. In like manner, there are those who either think that if they simply live a good and honorable life, the idea of balancing the figurative scales of justice, that this will ensure their entrance into heaven. While you did have in the Old Testament instances of individuals becoming servants of those with whom they had become debtors, but that doesn't work for the debt of sin. The Bible makes this point clear, James 2:10 says, "For whoever shall keep the whole law, and yet stumble in one point, he is guilty of all." Then others think that they have blown it so bad and that the price is too steep, that they see no way of getting out of spiritual debt. Somewhere along life's journey, the guilt of poor life-choices became so heavy that they became blind to the light of the Gospel. In both instances, this is true, the debt is too steep for anyone to attempt to repay and the bondage of guilt so debilitating that the Good News has been obscured. There are no human remedies for removing the stain and debt of sin. No being a better person, for there is none righteous (Romans 3:10), nor can we pretend that sin doesn't exist by playing ignorance, God requires repentance (Acts 17:30). With that being said, we also do not need to bound by the weight of guilt from our sins either because we have a Champion who came to set us free.

In the final moments of Jesus' life here on Earth, he proclaimed three final words, "It is finished" (John 19:30), and in so doing accomplished that for which the Father sent Him. This phrase has two primary applications, the first as was previously suggested, to fulfill a task or command of which Jesus spoke of in John 9:4, "I must work the works of Him who sent Me while it is day; the night is coming when no one can work." However, the other application is the one most interest to us as it part that made us free indeed, and that is in Jesus substituting Himself in our place, satisfied the justice of God in paying off our debt in full to which can never be revisited. In the Old Testament, when there was a debt that needed to pay an individual would go to work for the one the payment was due. But in the seventh year, seven being the number of perfection and/or competition, the debtor would be released from their debt, this was known as the "Year of Jubilee (Leviticus 25:39-43). Jesus' death on the cross, being both perfect and bringing complete restoration, paid off our spiritual credit card that was maxed out, thus removing our guilt, and His resurrection becomes our receipt of said payment. Thereby bringing with this freedom, our year of Jubilee. That is the essence of the Good News. The guilt that we have been dragging around has been wiped out, we no longer must live in bondage to bad life-choices and mistakes from the past because Jesus took care of it and it will never be looked at again. Isaiah 43:25 says, "I, even I, am He who blots out your transgressions for My own sake; And I will not remember your sins." Jesus is the ultimate chain breaker, releasing freedom from the guilt of sin, and replaces it with adoption into the family of God.

> *"It is the truth of grace and not of the law that brings you true freedom. The truth of the law only binds you. In fact, religious bondage is one of the most crippling bondages with which a person can be encumbered. Religious bondage keeps one in constant fear, guilt, and anxiety."*
> Joseph Prince

Condemnation

"Jesus Himself has already paid the price for your sins, so stop condemning yourself! Today, when you look into the mirror, what do you see? Do you see yourself trapped in all your failings, mistakes, and sins? Or do you see what God sees? My dear friend, when God sees you today, He sees Jesus. Use your eyes of faith and believe that as Jesus is, so are you. In God's eyes, you are righteous, you are favored, you are blessed, and you are healed. You are freed from all sin, all pangs of guilt, all forms of condemnation, and every bondage of addiction!"
Joseph Prince

Romans 8:1-2, "There is therefore now no condemnation to those who are in Christ Jesus, who do not walk according to the flesh, but according to the Spirit. For the law of the Spirit of life in Christ Jesus has made me free from the law of sin and death." Condemnation, according to Strong's, means the sentence pronounced," with a suggestion of the punishment following the pronouncement. Paul uses the Law as the backdrop to justify condemning a person, as unless one fulfills every aspect of the Law of God perfectly, then they violate defiling the whole Law, and in many cases the penalty was death. This is also why God instituted animal sacrifices as a substitute for the atonement of violating the Law. The animal had to be spotless and without blemish, such as a lamb, to be acceptable to God, and yet even this was a temporary covering, not a complete cleansing. The writer of Hebrews highlights this point, 10:11, "And every priest stands to minister daily and offering repeatedly the same sacrifices, which can never take away sins." As glorious as the Law was (2 Corinthians 3), it could never fully satisfy the righteous judgments of the Lord by human efforts. But praise is to the God of grace and mercy for sending someone who could satisfy the Law's requirements, namely The Anointed One, Yeshua Hamashiach. If only we would get out of our heads long enough to receive the freedom that this Good News brings.

Unfortunately, many of us because of guilt and shame, proclaim self-condemnation upon ourselves. It a good thing when conviction comes upon a person because they recognize that their thoughts or actions violate the relationship that we now enjoy with and through Jesus. There are many instances in the Bible of individuals acknowledging their sinful acts against the Lord and accepting responsibility for them. Probably one of, if not the most famous one is when the Prophet Nathan called out David's sin with Bathsheba, 2 Samuel 12:12-13, "For you did it secretly, but I will do this thing before all Israel, before the sun.' " So, David said to Nathan, "I have sinned against the Lord," revisited by David in Psalm 51. In my line of work, one of the first things that I encourage others to do to begin to make the necessary changes needed to improve overall health, sobriety, and quality of life is to acknowledge the mistakes made and then make amends for the poor life-choices. However, it is a whole other level to become stuck in a place of perpetual torment over mistakes, thinking that this is all that life has for us now, that I have blown it beyond any possible repair. All of which are brought about by fear, doubt, and lack of faith that the God who spoke the universe into existence cannot fix in us what we have done to ourselves, and perhaps there is some truth there in terms of the old covenant, but it certainly is not the case with the new covenant. And yet, this is the state of many who have walked away from the faith because of this line of thinking that God wouldn't want me anymore. The way that this occurs is in two ways, by others casting virtual stones at us, guilting and shaming us for our poor choices or decisions. Then there is the other, false humility. That is, by constantly degrading ourselves because, in our minds, we are somehow not worthy of accepting credit for the blessings and giftings of the Lord outwardly. Let us deal with stone-throwers first.

I think we all can think of moments in our lives where we feel as if we have blown it. That seemingly is the theme of life itself, and as I once heard Sylvester Stallone mention about one of the life lessons in the Rocky series. Life knocks us down, and many times it is a result of poor choices we've made. However, continuing the rocky theme, it isn't how many times life knocks you down, but how many times you get up. The problem comes from people in our lives who beat us up for the decisions we've made that resulted in the bad situations we find ourselves and are especially damaging when it comes to those closest to us. I know in my own life, it has happened to me and could have derailed my journey to becoming sober. It was June of 1995 when the Lord first visited me and essentially said: "You are done with these drugs." I had never had that type of experience before, heck I wasn't even walking with the Lord at this time. The only thing I knew was that something deep within me was compelled to rid myself of any resemblance of drugs, and then to share this news with my family thinking that they would be happy and supportive. I was wrong. I reply that I got was this, "You'll never do it." Wow! Why would they say that? Simple, because that is all that they saw me do is the drugs, and therefore couldn't fathom the thought that I could be strong enough or capable enough to succeed, and this is the story from many who have marks from the stones cast their way, that they are not smart enough, strong enough, capable enough, or good enough to overcome great difficulties to succeed until this becomes their truth. I have met many who struggled with the condemnation from others until they believed it themselves.

Imagine if Thomas Edison believed the people in his life who said that he wasn't smart enough to learn anything, maybe we have electricity later or maybe not. Now imagine this happening to people who are seeking the Church to be the support system that they need to be successful and to overcome adversity because their own families have stoned them. Unfortunately, it happens more times then we would like to acknowledge. The "religious" people are often guilty of injuring their own. So, how much do we suppose that they are more likely to reject someone who comes with baggage? There is this expression that goes "Don't throw stones when you live in a glasshouse," and Jesus also warned about throwing stones at other people, "He who is without sin among you, let him throw a stone at her first" (John 8:7). Paul also warned about casting stones at those outside the Church in 1 Corinthians 5, "For what have I to do with judging those also who are outside?" (v.12). Paul goes on to say examine yourself and those inside the body of Christ, and yet we eat our won just as bad even though Paul admonishes us to "restore such a one in a spirit of gentleness, considering yourself lest you also be tempted" (Galatians 6:1). So, back to my family's appraisal of me. Well, I could have caved to their low opinion of me and believed that I was doomed to be an addict for the rest of my life, condemned to a life of torment. I mean maybe I wasn't strong enough, good enough, or capable enough to overcome these poor life-choices. Truth is, almost 25 years later, I keep those stones with me as a reminder of the fact that by the grace and mercy of God, I was strong enough, good enough, or capable enough to overcome those poor life-choices, but there are those out there despite getting the victory, diminish the work of God in them with false-humility.

False humility in spiritual circles is often promoted with the passage "He must increase, but I must decrease," (John 3:30). The notion is never taking credit for anything and simply saying "It wasn't me but God," and while in the grand scheme of things this may be true, the fact is that this type of humility is pride in disguise. It is beating one's self up to avoid becoming prideful, imposing rules and standards upon self to deny any indication of arrogance. The problem is that the focus has turned from the Lord to the rejection of self, which then becomes a form of pride, religion, and idol worship. The Bible speaks about this very clearly. Colossians 2:20-23 says, "Therefore, if you died with Christ from the basic principles of the world, why, as though living in the world, do you subject yourselves to regulations— "Do not touch, do not taste, do not handle," which all concern things which perish with the using— according to the commandments and doctrines of men? These things indeed have an appearance of wisdom in self-imposed religion, false humility, and neglect of the body, but are of no value against the indulgence of the flesh." While the passage here references those attempting to keep the Law of God, the principle is relevant, self-imposed denial and punishments despite the old covenant being replaced for the new covenant. Subjecting ourselves to man-made religious rules and regulations is an afront to the freedom that the Lord purchased by His blood for us. It a self-imposed condemnation for the inability to abstain from this, that, or the other thing rather than living in the perfect liberty of Christ. Ultimately, it becomes devotion to the sacrifice of self over the sacrifice of Jesus, it is trying to justify self which ends in condemnation, and that is pride, not humility. Remember Romans 8:1, "There is therefore now no condemnation to those who are in Christ Jesus, who do not walk according to the flesh, but according to the Spirit."

"What ground is left for accusation since sin's penalty has been fully paid? The blood of the Lord has atoned for all the sins of a believer; hence there is no more condemnation in the conscience." Watchman Nee

Summary:

Final Thought

They say that the hardest prison to gain freedom from is the prison within which many have sentenced themselves to be condemned for poor life-choices or the abuses imposed by others, and this does not have to be a life sentence. Everyday work with individuals who are in the criminal system and will eventually be sent to prison for mistakes that they have made. However, these individuals will eventually be released from prison and hopefully, begin a new life having learned from their mistakes. Jesus came, according to Luke 4:18, to "preach the gospel to the poor; He has sent Me to heal the brokenhearted, To proclaim liberty to the captives And recovery of sight to the blind, To set at liberty those who are oppressed; To proclaim the acceptable year of the Lord." The gospel is set to heal those poor in spirit, brokenhearted by the decisions they have made and rejection of others because of those choices, and to release us from the prison of torment and shame that sin imposes on us. To set at liberty anyone who calls on the name of the Lord from the prison within. If this is something that you struggle with as much as I still do, then RIGHT NOW, pause and ask the Lord to reveal the source and proclaim peace and freedom to that area of your life, and watch the Lord free you from yourself. YOU are good enough, strong enough, capable enough, and loved enough to realize this victory because Jesus has already claimed it for you.

> *"Jesus allows Himself to be bound, because His bonds are to break the chains of our sins. Jesus becomes a slave for our sakes, through the excess of His charity alone, to free our souls from the slavery of the devil. Offer yourself to Him now, to be entirely His, beseeching Him to bind you fast with the sweet chains of His love."* Ignatius of the Side of Jesus Passionist

Bibliography

"BibleGateway." BibleGateway.com: A Searchable Online Bible in over 150 Versions and 50 Languages., 29 Sept. 2019, https://www.biblegateway.com/.

"Blue Letter Bible." Blue Letter Bible - Home Page, 29 Sept. 2019, http://www.blbclassic.org/.

Boom, Corrie Ten. "Clippings from My Notebook: Writings and Sayings Collected." Amazon, World Wide Publications, 1984, https://www.amazon.com/Clippings-Notebook-Corrie-Ten-Boom/dp/0840741022.

BOUNDS, EDWARD M. PURPOSE IN PRAYER. WILDER PUBLICATIONS, 2018.

"Catholic Treasury: The Dialogue of St Catherine of Siena." Catholic Treasury | The Dialogue of St Catherine of Siena, http://www.catholictreasury.info/books/dialogue/index.php.

Chantry, Walter J. "The Shadow of the Cross: Studies in Self-Denial." Amazon, Banner of Truth Trust, 1981, https://www.amazon.com/Shadow-Cross-Studies-Self-Denial/dp/085151331X.

Dawkins, Robbie. "Do What Jesus Did: A Real-Life Field Guide to Healing the Sick, Routing Demons, and Changing Lives Forever." Robby Dawkins: 9780800795573 - Christianbook.com, Chosen Books, https://www.christianbook.com/healing-routing-demons-changing-lives-forever/robby-dawkins/9780800795573/pd/795573.

Elliot, Elisabeth. Through Gates of Splendor. Hendrickson Publishers, 2015.

Frangipane, Francis. The Three Battlegrounds. Arrow Publications, 2006.

Gilbert, Elizabeth. Eat, Pray, Love: One Womans Search for Everything across Italy, India and Indonesia. Riverhead Books, 2017.

Hammond, Michelle McKinney. "Release the Pain, Embrace the Joy." Amazon, Regal Books, 2005, https://www.amazon.com/Release-Embrace-Michelle-McKinney-Hammond/dp/0764214780.

Ignatius of St. Paul of the side of Jesus. The School of Jesus Crucified, from the Italian of Father Ignatius of the Side of Jesus, Passionist. Burns Oates & Washbourne Ltd., 1922.

Johnson, Bill. "When Heaven Invades Earth: a Practical Guide to a Life of Miracles." Amazon, Destiny Image Publishers, 2013, https://www.amazon.com/When-Heaven-Invades-Earth-Devotional/dp/0768422973.

Keller, Timothy. The Reason for God Belief in an Age of Skepticism. Riverhead Books, 2009.

Kroll, Woodrow. Lessons on Living from Job: a Devotional. Back to the Bible Publishing, 1999.

Luis. The Sinners Guide from Vice to Virtue; Giving Him Instructions and Directions How to Become Virtuous. Translated from the Spanish of Lewis of Granada. Printed for M. Cooper, 1761.

Meyer, F. B. Our Daily Walk. Marshall, Morgan & Scott, 1951.

MOODY, DWIGHT L. SECRET POWER: the Secret of Success in Christian Life and Work. ANEKO Press, 2017.

Moore, Beth. Breaking Free Discover the Victory of Total Surrender. B & H Publishing Group, 2014.

"Most Teenagers Drop Out of Church as Young Adults." LifeWay Research, 16 Jan. 2019, https://lifewayresearch.com/2019/01/15/most-teenagers-drop-out-of-church-as-young-adults/.

Murdock, Mike. The Law of Recognition: Discovering the Gifts, Opportunities & Relationships That God Has Already Placed in Your Life. Wisdom International, 2007.

Nee, Watchman. The Spiritual Man. Christian Fellowship Pub., 1977.

ORR, JAMES. INTERNATIONAL STANDARD BIBLE ENCYCLOPAEDIA: Naarah-Socho (Classic Reprint). FORGOTTEN Books, 2017.

Ortberg, John. Soul Keeping: Caring for the Most Important Part of You. Zondervan, 2014.

Prince, Joseph. "The Power of Right Believing: 7 Keys to Freedom from Fear, Guilt, and Addiction." Amazon, Faithwords, 2013, https://www.amazon.com/Power-Right-Believing-Freedom-Addiction/dp/1455553166.

Russell, Jesse, and Ronald Cohn. Strongs Concordance. LENNEX Corp, 2012.

SENECA, LUCIUS ANNAEUS. Senecas Morals of a Happy Life, Benefits, Anger and Clemency. ECHO LIBRARY, 2017.

Simpson, Albert Benjamin. Days of Heaven upon Earth. Christianalliance, 1897.

Solomon, Joseph. "A Shadow of a Doubt." A Shadow of a Doubt. 26 Apr. 2014, Houston.

Sproul, R. C. Faith Alone: the Evangelical Doctrine of Justification. Baker Books, 2017.

SPURGEON, CHARLES HADDON. SERMONS OF REV. C.H. SPURGEON OF LONDON. FORGOTTEN Books, 2015.

Stanley, Charles F. Man of God: Leading Your Family by Allowing God to Lead You. David C Cook, 2015.

Tada, Joni Eareckson. Is God Really in Control? Joni and Friends, 1990.

Wiersbe, Warren W. The Strategy of Satan How to Detect & Defeat Him. Tyndale House Publishers, Inc., 2011.

Wilberforce, William. Real Christianity. Barbour Pub., 1999.